Home Rehabilitation Exercises

Hand

Kay Lee, OTR
Shirley Marcus, OTR

Illustrations by Dan Winter

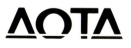

The American Occupational Therapy Association, Inc.
Rockville, Maryland

It is the objective of the American Occupational Therapy Association to be a
forum for free expression and interchange of ideas. The opinions and
positions expressed by contributors to this work are their own and not
necessarily those of either the editors or the American Occupational Therapy
Association, Inc.

The exercises in this book must be performed under the supervision of a
therapist or physician, and the authors disclaim any liability in the event of
an inappropriate use of the exercises that leads to injury.

This publication is available in a Spanish-language edition.

The American Occupational Therapy Association, Inc.
1383 Piccard Drive, PO Box 1725
Rockville, MD 20849-1725
(301) 948-9626, Fax (301) 948-5512, TDD (1-800) 377-8555

Director of Publications: Anne E. Rosenstein

Editor: Duncan Clark

Cover Design: Robert Sacheli

5,3
3
70

Information to Remember

Doctor's name and phone number:

_____

_____

Occupational therapist's name and phone number:

_____

_____

IMPORTANT: These are your precautions. If you have any questions or problems, contact your doctor or therapist.

_____

_____

_____

_____

_____

_____

_____

_____

_____

To The Patient

Range of motion is the amount of free movement available at any particular joint. When joints are not moved, they become stiff and painful. Repetitive movement through the fullest possible range prevents these problems. You can make sure your joints move freely, even if your arm or hand is weak, by following the exercises in this booklet and repeating them **as instructed by your physician or therapist.**

Principles of Range of Motion Exercises

1. Establish a daily routine for performing exercises. Your therapist or physician will advise you as to how many times per day you should exercise and how many repetitions per session. If you have no other guidelines, you should exercise 3 sessions per day; start with 5 repetitions of each movement (holding each position for a count of 5) and work up to 10 repetitions.

2. Move the joint as far as possible *without forcing* the joint beyond its range.

3. Always stretch *gently.* Stretches should be long and slow. **DO NOT BOUNCE!** You should feel a stretch but *not pain.*

4. Remember to breathe while exercising.

5. Relax between exercises.

6. Exercise fingers individually, then as a group.

7. Always stabilize the joints below the one(s) you are working on.

8. **For your protection, review these exercises with your therapist or physician prior to use.** It is imperative that they are performed correctly and under professional supervision.

9. If your exercises produce pain or swelling later in the day, consult your therapist or physician immediately.

Basic Anatomy of the Hand

Thumb:

IP - Interphalangeal joint
MP - Metacarpophalangeal joint

Fingers:

DIP - Distal interphalangeal joints
PIP - Proximal interphalangeal joints
MP - Metacarpophalangeal joints

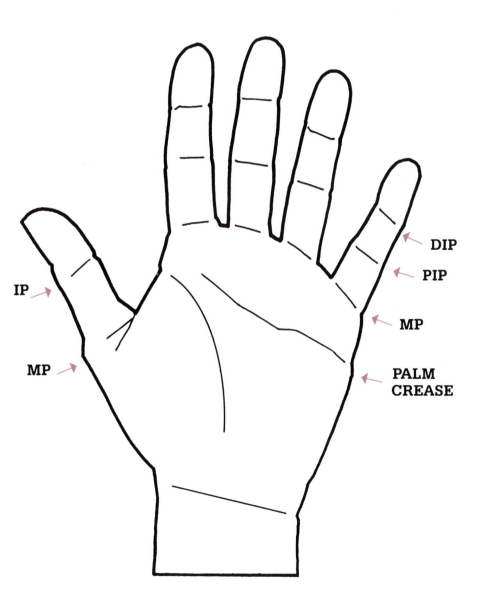

Active Thumb MP
Flexion and Extension

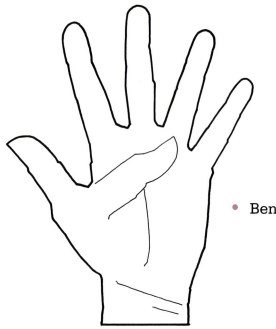

• Bend and straighten **MP** joint.

Thumb MP Flexion and
Extension Stretch

• Bend **MP** while stretching with
  other hand.

• Hold thumb position and
  remove other hand.

• Straighten thumb.

• Stretch straight with other hand.

• Hold thumb position and
  remove other hand.

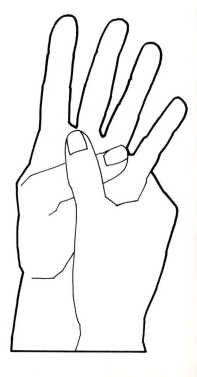

Active Thumb IP Flexion and Extension

- Bend and straighten thumb tip at **IP** joint.

Thumb IP Flexion and Extension Stretch

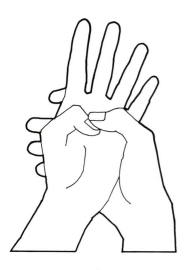

- Bend thumb tip (**IP**) while stretching with other hand.

- Hold thumb position and remove other hand.

- Straighten thumb.

- Stretch **IP** joint straight with other hand.

- Hold thumb position and remove other hand.

Blocked IP Flexion and Active Extension

- Block **MP** joint with other hand.

- Bend and straighten thumb tip at **IP** joint.

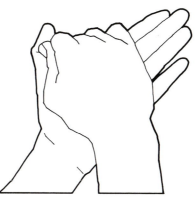

Active Composite Thumb Flexion/Extension

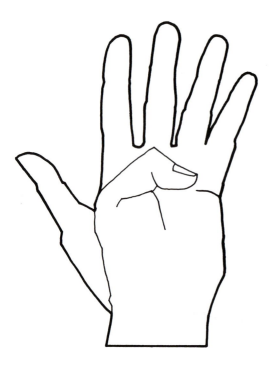

- Bend thumb tip **(IP)** to base of little finger at crease.

- Straighten thumb completely.

Composite Thumb Flexion/Extension Stretch

- Stretch thumb tip **(IP)** to palm crease with other hand.

- Hold position and remove other hand.

- Straighten thumb completely.

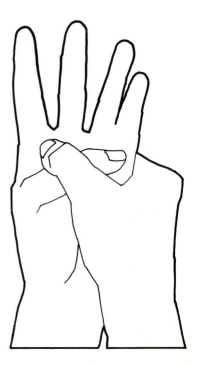

Active Radial Abduction

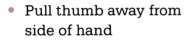

- Pull thumb away from side of hand

Active Thumb Palmar Abduction/Adduction

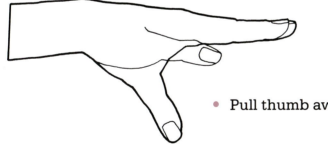

- Pull thumb away from palm.

Active Opposition

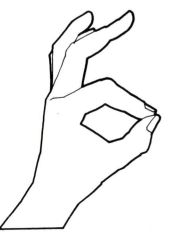

- Touch thumb tip to each fingertip alternately.

Active MP Flexion and Extension

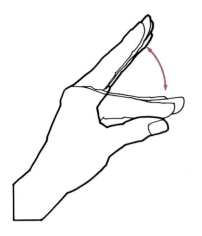

- Bend **MPs** with **IPs** straight.
- Straighten **MPs** with **IPs** straight.

MP Flexion and Extension Stretch

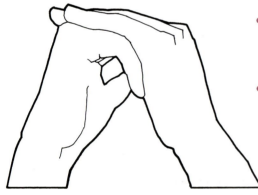

- Bend **MPs** while stretching with other hand.
- Hold position and remove other hand.

- Stretch **MPs** in straight position using other hand.
- Hold position and remove other hand.

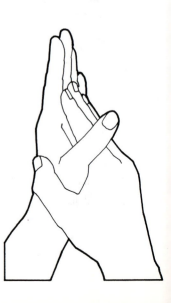

Active PIP Flexion and Extension

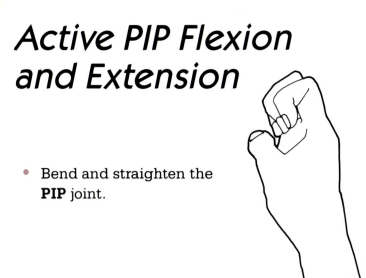

- Bend and straighten the **PIP** joint.

PIP Flexion and Extension Stretch

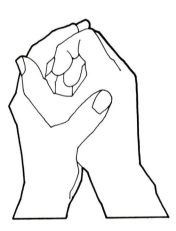

- Bend **PIP** while stretching with other hand.
- Hold position and release other hand.
- Straighten **PIP.**
- Stretch in straight position using other hand.
- Hold position and remove other hand.

Blocked PIP Flexion and Active Extension

- Block motion at the **MP** joint.
- Bend and straighten at the **PIP** joint.

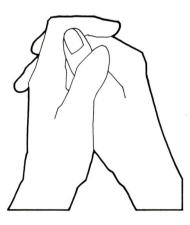

DIP Flexion and Extension Stretch

- Bend **DIP** and **PIP** while stretching with other hand.

- Hold position and remove other hand.

- *Caution: Do not stretch **DIP** too forcefully.*

- Straighten **DIP.**

- Using other hand, stretch to straighten completely.

- Hold.

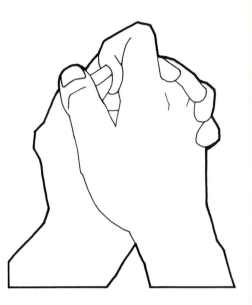

Blocked DIP Flexion and Active Extension

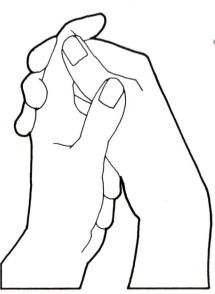

- Block **PIP** and **MP** with other hand.

- Bend and straighten at **DIP.**

Active Composite Flexion and Extension

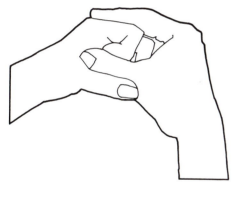

- Make a fist.
- Open the hand.

Composite Flexion and Extension Stretch

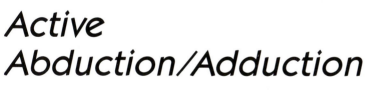

- Make a fist.
- Stretch each finger to curl towards palm.
- Hold position.
- Straighten fingers completely.

Active Abduction/Adduction

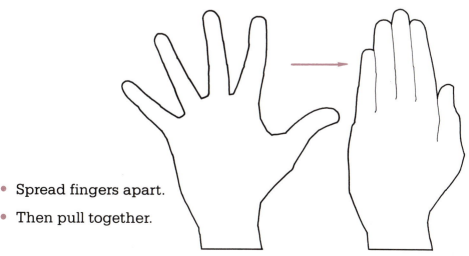

- Spread fingers apart.
- Then pull together.

Intrinsic Minus/Plus Positions

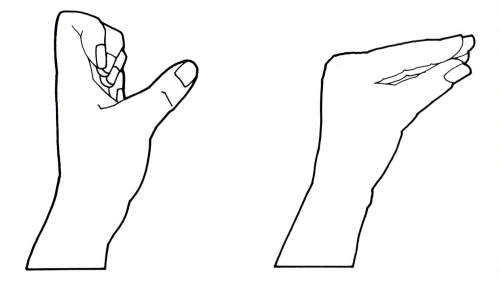

- Straighten **MPs** and curl both **PIPs** and **DIPs**.
- Then bend **MPs** and straighten **PIPs** and **DIPs**.

Intrinsic Stretch

- Straighten **MPs**, curl **PIPs** and **DIPs** into the "hook" position.
- Gently stretch with other hand.
- Hold position and remove other hand.

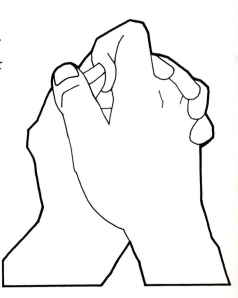

Tendon Glide

- Begin in straight position, roll into hook position, bending **DIPs** and **PIPs**. Return to straight.
- Begin in straight position, roll into fist, bending **MPs, PIPs,** and **DIPs.** Return to straight.
- Begin in straight position, roll into straight fist, bending **MPs** and **PIPs** (keeping **DIPs** straight). Return to straight.

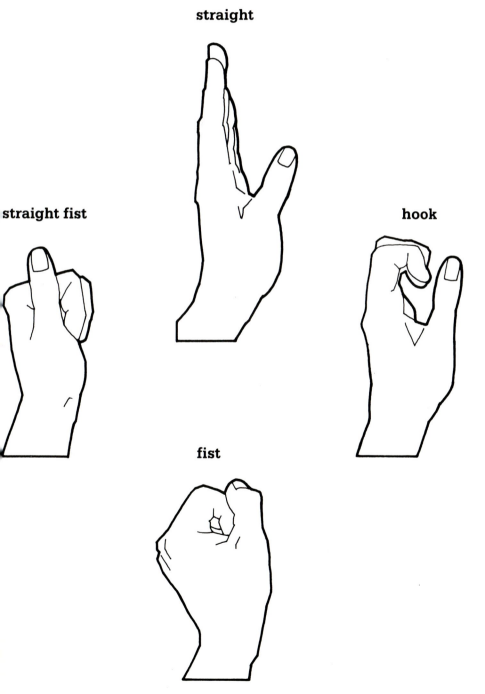

straight

straight fist

hook

fist

Specific recommendations for you:

_____

_____

_____

_____

_____

_____

_____

_____

_____

_____

_____

_____

_____

_____

_____

_____

_____

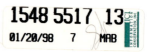

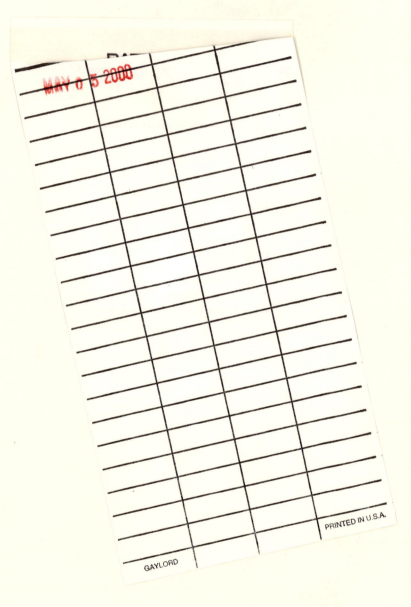